STAGE 5 KIDNEY DISEASE DIET COOKBOOK FOR SENIORS

Nutritious and Delicious Recipes with Low Sodium, Potassium, and Phosphorus for Effective Meal Planning in Managing Chronic Kidney Disease.

Richie Smile Walker

Copyright © 2024 **Richie Smile Walker**

All Rights Are Reserved

The content in this book may not be reproduced, duplicated, or transferred without the express written permission of the author or publisher. Under no circumstances will the publisher or author be held liable or legally responsible for any losses, expenditures, or damages incurred directly or indirectly as a consequence of the information included in this book.

Legal Remarks

Copyright protection applies to this publication. It is only intended for personal use. No piece of this work may be modified, distributed, sold, quoted, or paraphrased without the author's or publisher's consent.

Disclaimer Statement

Please keep in mind that the contents of this booklet are meant for educational and recreational purposes. Every effort has been made to offer accurate, up-to-date, reliable, and thorough information. There are, however, no stated or implied assurances of any kind. Readers understand that the author is providing competent counsel. The content in this book originates from several sources. Please seek the opinion of a competent professional before using any of the tactics outlined in this book. By reading this book, the reader agrees that the author will not be held accountable for any direct or indirect damages resulting from the use of the information contained therein, including, but not limited to, errors, omissions, or inaccuracies.

TABLE OF CONTENTS

INTRODUCTION **6**
   Understanding Stage 5 Kidney Disease 7
   Causes of stage 5 kidney disease in Seniors........................11

CHAPTER 1 ....**15**
DIETARY BASICS FOR STAGE 5 KIDNEY DISEASE **15**
   Nutritional Needs and Restrictions..................................15
   Potassium, Phosphorus, and Sodium: Balancing Act................17
   The Role of Protein: Quality Over Quantity 20
   Reading Food Labels: What to Look For 23

CHAPTER 2 ....**26**
BREAKFAST RECIPES...**26**
   Apple-Cinnamon Oatmeal..26
   Low-Potassium Berry Smoothie 27
   Egg White Veggie Scramble 28
   Avocado Toast with Radishes 29
   Cottage Cheese with Pineapple 31
   Almond Butter Banana Smoothie.....................................32
   Chia Seed Pudding 33
   Turkey and Spinach Omelet 34
   Quinoa Breakfast Bowl 35
   Ricotta and Honey Toast 36

CHAPTER 3 ....**38**
LUNCH RECIPES...**38**
   Tuna Salad Stuffed Avocado..38
   Chickpea Greek Salad 39

Vegetable Lentil Soup 41
Quinoa Chicken Salad 42
Turkey Wrap with Cranberry and Spinach 43
Mediterranean Chickpea Salad 45
Roasted Vegetable Quiche 46
Cold Pasta Salad with Tuna 47
Chicken Avocado Wrap 49
Beet and Goat Cheese Salad 50

CHAPTER 4 52
DINNER RECIPES 52

Baked Lemon Herb Chicken 52
One-Pot Vegetable Pasta 53
Grilled Salmon with Dill Yogurt Sauce 55
Stuffed Bell Peppers 56
Roasted Chicken and Vegetables 58
Herb-crusted cod with Asparagus 59
Vegetarian Stuffed Zucchini Boats 60
Lemon Garlic Shrimp with Broccoli 62
Turkey and Sweet Potato Skillet 63
Grilled Vegetable Platter with Herb Drizzle 65

CHAPTER 5 67
SNACKS AND DESSERTS 67

Apple Cinnamon Chips 67
Rice Cake with Avocado and Tomato 68
Chilled Berry Soup 69
Peanut Butter Banana Bites 70
Vanilla Almond Mousse 71
Cucumber Hummus Bites 73

Carrot Cake Oatmeal Cookies 74
Frozen Yogurt Bark 75
Zucchini Bread Muffins 76
Peach Sorbet 78

CHAPTER 6 80
BEVERAGES AND SMOOTHIES 80
Cucumber Mint Water 80
Berry Blast Kidney-Friendly Smoothie 81
Chamomile Lavender Tea 82
Green Detox Smoothie 83
Ginger Pear Infusion 84
Watermelon Cucumber Slush 85
Almond Milk Matcha Latte 87
Pineapple Coconut Water Smoothie 88
Herbal Berry Iced Tea 89
Golden Milk Turmeric Tea 90

CHAPTER 7 92
MEAL PLAN 92
Frequently asked questions 99

CHAPTER 8 102
CONCLUSION 102

INTRODUCTION

"Food is not just sustenance, but medicine, comfort, and a way to connect with others. In the journey of managing Stage 5 Kidney Disease, it becomes a beacon of hope and a path to wellness."

Journeying through the complexities of Stage 5 Kidney Disease, especially in the golden years, presents a unique set of challenges and opportunities. The diagnosis, while daunting, opens a door to a deeper understanding of the profound impact that diet and nutrition have on our well-being. This cookbook is not just a collection of recipes; it's a guide, a companion, and a source of inspiration for seniors and their families who are on this journey.

The essence of managing kidney disease at this stage lies in the delicate balance of nutrients, the understanding of what the body needs, and how to provide it without overwhelming compromised kidneys. It's about making informed choices that nourish the body, cater to the palate, and respect the limitations imposed by this condition. This task, while seemingly Herculean, is made approachable and achievable through the pages of this book.

We embark on this journey with a spirit of empathy and empowerment, recognizing the individual struggles and victories that come with dietary management of kidney disease. The goal is not to dwell on the restrictions but to celebrate the possibilities. Through carefully crafted recipes, practical advice, and nutritional insights, we aim to illuminate the path to a fulfilling and flavorful dietary regimen that supports kidney health and enhances the quality of life.

This book is a testament to the resilience of the human spirit and the healing power of food. It is designed to encourage exploration, experimentation, and enjoyment in eating, all while safeguarding kidney function and promoting overall health. Whether you're a senior navigating the complexities of Stage 5 Kidney Disease, a caregiver seeking to provide the best care, or simply someone looking to understand more about this condition, this cookbook offers strategies for improvement, a dose of inspiration, and a way forward.

Let us journey together through the pages of this cookbook, discovering not just recipes, but a new perspective on food, health, and the joy of eating well with kidney disease. Welcome to a world where every meal is an opportunity for nourishment, comfort, and celebration.

Understanding Stage 5 Kidney Disease

In the realm of health and wellness, few diagnoses are as impactful as that of Stage 5 Kidney Disease. This condition, often the culmination of a gradual decline in kidney function, marks a significant shift in how one approaches life, diet, and overall health management. It's a moment that calls for reflection, education, and adaptation, not just for those diagnosed but also for their families and caregivers.

The Essence of Stage 5 Kidney Disease

At its core, Stage 5 Kidney Disease, also known as End-Stage Renal Disease (ESRD), is characterized by the near or complete failure of kidney function. The kidneys, those vital organs responsible for filtering waste and excess fluids from the blood, lose their ability to perform this crucial task effectively. The implications of this are profound, affecting every aspect of an individual's health and daily living.

Understanding this condition begins with recognizing its signs and symptoms, which can include fatigue, fluid retention, nausea, a decrease in urine output, and difficulties in concentration. These symptoms are not just indicators of the disease's presence but also a call to action for a more managed and mindful approach to health.

The Impact on Daily Life

The transition to living with Stage 5 Kidney Disease is profound. It necessitates a reevaluation of one's lifestyle, particularly in the areas of diet and nutrition. The foods and beverages that were once staples of one's diet may now need to be reconsidered or replaced. This is not about restriction but rather about transformation. It's about finding new ways to enjoy food while respecting the body's changed needs.

Moreover, treatment options such as dialysis become a significant part of life. These treatments, while life-sustaining, also bring their own set of challenges and adjustments. They require time, patience, and resilience, both from the individual undergoing treatment and their support network.

A Path Forward

The diagnosis of Stage 5 Kidney Disease is undeniably challenging, but it also opens up a pathway to resilience and empowerment. Education plays a pivotal role in this journey. Understanding the intricacies of the disease, from its effects on the body to how diet and lifestyle can mitigate these impacts, is crucial. It equips individuals and their families with the knowledge needed to make informed decisions about their care and well-being.

This knowledge also fosters a sense of control and agency. In a situation where so much can feel uncertain, having clear, actionable information about how to manage one's health can be incredibly empowering. It's about shifting the narrative from one of limitation to one of possibility.

The Role of Diet in Managing Stage 5 Kidney Disease

Dietary management becomes a cornerstone of living with Stage 5 Kidney Disease. The right diet can help manage symptoms, reduce the burden on the kidneys, and improve quality of life. This involves a careful balance of nutrients, mindful of the kidneys' reduced capacity to filter and eliminate waste products from the body.

Protein, potassium, phosphorus, and sodium are among the nutrients that require careful monitoring. The goal is to prevent the accumulation of waste products in the blood while ensuring that the body receives the nutrition it needs to function optimally. This delicate balance is not about deprivation but about making choices that support kidney health and overall well-being.

Embracing Support and Community

No one should navigate the complexities of Stage 5 Kidney Disease alone. Support from healthcare professionals, dietitians, family, and friends plays an invaluable role in managing this condition. These support networks provide not just practical assistance but also emotional support, understanding, and encouragement.

Moreover, connecting with others who are on a similar journey can be incredibly affirming. It offers a sense of community and shared experience, reminding individuals that they are not alone in their challenges. These connections can also be a source of practical advice, tips, and recipes that can make managing the dietary aspects of the disease more manageable and enjoyable.

Reflection and Adaptation

Living with Stage 5 Kidney Disease is undeniably a profound adjustment. It requires a reevaluation of one's lifestyle, priorities, and approach to health. Yet, within this challenge lies an opportunity for growth, resilience, and a deeper appreciation for the role of diet and lifestyle in managing chronic conditions.

This chapter of life, though marked by change, is also filled with possibilities. It's an invitation to embrace a more mindful and nourished way of living, to discover new flavors and foods that support health, and to connect with others on a similar path. It's a journey of adaptation, learning, and, ultimately, empowerment.

Causes of stage 5 kidney disease in Seniors

In the golden years of life, when wisdom flourishes and stories abound, health becomes a canvas of lived experiences, each brushstroke marked by choices, challenges, and sometimes, the unforeseen forces of nature. Among the myriad health challenges that may emerge, Stage 5 Kidney Disease stands as a sentinel, reminding us of the delicate balance our bodies navigate daily. Understanding the causes of this profound condition is not just an exercise in medical literacy; it's a journey into the heart of our collective resilience and the quest for wellness that defines the human spirit.

The Culprits Unmasked

At the core of Stage 5 Kidney Disease in seniors are several key factors, each contributing in its way to the progression of this condition. These factors are not merely clinical observations but narratives of how our bodies, environment, and choices intertwine, shaping our health landscapes.

1. The Legacy of Chronic Conditions

Chronic diseases, like hypertension and diabetes, are the twin colossi standing at the forefront of kidney disease causes. Hypertension, with its silent, insidious nature, escalates the wear and tear on the delicate blood vessels of the kidneys. Diabetes, on the other hand, casts a long shadow through high blood sugar levels, which can damage the kidneys' intricate filtering system over time. These conditions, prevalent in the tapestry of senior health, underscore the interconnectedness of bodily systems and the ripple effects of chronic disease management.

2. The Age Factor

Aging, in its natural progression, brings about changes in kidney structure and function. The kidneys' filtering units, the nephrons, diminish in number and efficiency, a testament to the passage of time. This decline is a natural aspect of aging, yet when coupled with other risk factors, it accelerates the journey toward kidney disease. It's a reminder of the body's finite resilience and the importance of nurturing it through every season of life.

3. The Shadow of Autoimmune Diseases

Autoimmune diseases, where the body's immune system turns against its tissues, can target the kidneys in a mistaken assault. Conditions like lupus nephritis embody this internal strife, marking a path of inflammation and damage that can culminate in Stage 5 Kidney Disease. These diseases speak to the complexity of the body's defense mechanisms and the fine line they tread between protection and harm.

4. The Impact of Obstructions and Infections

Urinary tract obstructions and repeated kidney infections carve a path of scarring and damage, leading to a decline in kidney function. These conditions, often marked by pain and discomfort, highlight the vulnerability of the kidneys to external insults and the importance of addressing urinary health issues promptly and effectively.

5. The Role of Medications and Toxins

Certain medications, especially those used long-term for chronic conditions, can bear a heavy toll on the kidneys. Similarly, exposure to environmental toxins, including heavy metals and pollutants, can contribute to kidney damage. This aspect of kidney health illuminates the delicate balance between treatment and toxicity, and the need for vigilant, informed use of medications and awareness of environmental exposures.

Reflections on the Path Forward

Understanding the causes of Stage 5 Kidney Disease in seniors is not about assigning blame or dwelling on what might have been. It's about illuminating the path forward, armed with knowledge and a resolve to nurture our health with intention and care. It's a call to action for individuals and communities alike to advocate for preventive measures, early detection, and management of chronic conditions that can lead to kidney disease.

This journey of understanding also opens a dialogue about the value of comprehensive healthcare that views the individual as a whole, recognizing the interconnectedness of conditions like hypertension, diabetes, and kidney disease. It's a testament to the power of lifestyle choices, medical innovation, and community support in shaping health outcomes.

CHAPTER 1

DIETARY BASICS FOR STAGE 5 KIDNEY DISEASE

Nutritional Needs and Restrictions

When the journey of life meanders into the realm of Stage 5 Kidney Disease, especially in the golden years, the narrative around food and nutrition transforms. It becomes less about the mere act of eating and more about the art of choosing—each meal, each bite, a deliberate decision towards balance and health. This isn't just about following a list of dietary restrictions; it's about redefining our relationship with food, turning it into a source of healing and strength.

The Essence of Protein: A Delicate Balance

Protein, the building block of life, assumes a nuanced role in this chapter of our health story. The conventional wisdom of 'more is better' fades, giving way to a strategy of precision. High-quality protein sources, those that offer maximum benefit with minimal waste, become our allies. It's a shift towards consuming with purpose, where plant-based proteins and lean meats are not just food but medicine, aiding our body without overwhelming our kidneys.

Potassium and Phosphorus: The Invisible Lines

Potassium and phosphorus, omnipresent in many foods, now require a second glance. These minerals, once consumed without a second thought, now stand as markers of a dietary boundary. The art lies in moderation and informed choice, navigating the landscape of fruits, vegetables, and dairy with an eye toward potassium and phosphorus content. It's a subtle dance, balancing these essential nutrients to avoid the extremes of too much or too little.

Sodium: Redefining Flavor

Sodium, the culinary world's longstanding companion, now presents a challenge. Its pervasive presence in our diets, once benign, becomes a concern, urging a reevaluation of how we flavor our food. This constraint, however, opens the door to culinary creativity. Herbs, spices, and sodium-free seasonings emerge as the heroes of flavor, proving that a reduction in salt does not equate to a loss in taste.

Fluids: The Measure of Mindfulness

In the intricate ballet of managing Stage 5 Kidney Disease, fluid intake becomes a performance of precision. The balance of hydration and fluid restriction is a personal rhythm, unique to each individual's condition and needs. It's about mindfulness, measuring, and monitoring not just for the sake of adherence but for the harmony of our body's systems.

Guidance: The Compass of Care

Embarking on this nutritional journey without guidance is akin to navigating without a map. Dietitians and healthcare professionals become our compass, offering direction in a landscape that can often feel bewildering. Their expertise is not just in crafting meal plans but in teaching us how to make informed, healthful choices. They are the translators, turning the complex language of nutrition into actionable, everyday practices.

Food as a Journey, Not Just a Destination

This exploration into the nutritional needs and restrictions of Stage 5 Kidney Disease is more than a regimen; it's a journey of discovery. Food, in this context, becomes a canvas for creativity, a medium for expression, and a testament to resilience. It's about finding joy in the kitchen again, experimenting with flavors, and celebrating the meals that nourish not just our bodies but our spirits. Reflecting on our health and dietary choices becomes an act of self-care, a deliberate pause in the rush of life to consider what truly nourishes us. It's a commitment to living well, even within the confines of dietary restrictions, and a reminder that within every limitation lies the potential for innovation and joy

Potassium, Phosphorus, and Sodium: Balancing Act

In the theater of nutrition, especially for those navigating the complexities of Stage 5 Kidney Disease, three pivotal elements take center stage: potassium, phosphorus, and sodium. Their interplay is not just a subplot in the narrative of dietary management but a central theme, a balancing act that demands both science and art to navigate successfully. This chapter delves into the essence of these elements, unraveling their roles and guiding you through the delicate dance of maintaining equilibrium in a body that has unique nutritional needs.

Potassium: The Heart's Conductor

Potassium, a mineral revered for its role in maintaining cellular function and heart health, becomes a character of paradox in the context of kidney disease. Essential yet potentially perilous when kidneys falter, its management is akin to walking a tightrope. Too little, and the body's symphony of cellular functions descends into chaos; too much, and the heart, the maestro of our bodily orchestra, risks losing its rhythm.

The key lies in moderation and mindful selection. Fruits, vegetables, and whole grains, the traditional bearers of potassium, must be chosen with care, balancing nutritional needs with the imperative to avoid excess. The narrative shifts from abundance to precision, selecting foods that nourish without overburdening the kidneys' compromised ability to maintain potassium balance.

Phosphorus: The Shadow Dancer

Phosphorus, often dancing in the shadows, unnoticed, plays a critical role in bone health and energy production. Yet, in the realm of kidney disease, it emerges as a formidable challenge, a mineral that must be watched closely. Excess phosphorus, when not excreted efficiently by the kidneys, invites a cascade of complications, from bone disease to heart ailments, a reminder of the interconnectedness of our body's systems.

The strategy for managing phosphorus is twofold: dietary vigilance and the embrace of phosphorus binders, when necessary. Foods rich in phosphorus, including dairy products, nuts, and meats, require careful consideration, balancing their nutritional benefits against the risk of phosphorus accumulation. It's a nuanced approach, seeking harmony in the body's mineral composition without tipping the scales towards harm.

Sodium: The Flavor of Caution

Sodium, the architect of flavor in many a culinary creation, assumes a more complex role for those with Stage 5 Kidney Disease. Its pervasiveness in diets, particularly in processed foods, becomes a concern, necessitating a shift in how we season our meals. The challenge is not merely one of reduction but of reimagining flavor, exploring the bounty of herbs, spices, and sodium-free seasonings that can elevate a dish without elevating blood pressure or exacerbating fluid retention.

This reevaluation of sodium is not just about avoiding certain foods but about redefining our relationship with taste, discovering that the essence of flavor lies not in salt alone but in the myriad of tastes that food inherently offers. It's an invitation to culinary creativity, a journey towards finding joy in the flavors that nature provides, unmasked by excessive salt.

The Balancing Act: A Path Forward

Handling the balance of potassium, phosphorus, and sodium is not a solitary journey but a collaborative endeavor. It involves engaging with healthcare professionals, from nephrologists to dietitians, who can provide tailored advice and support. It's about equipping oneself with knowledge, understanding not just the "what" but the "why" behind each dietary choice, and recognizing the profound impact these choices have on health and well-being.

This balancing act is also a testament to the resilience of the human spirit, and the capacity to adapt and find balance even in the face of daunting challenges. It's about making informed choices, embracing change, and finding new ways to enjoy food and nourish the body.

Reflecting on the roles of potassium, phosphorus, and sodium in our diets invites a deeper appreciation for the complexity of our bodies and the foods that fuel them. It's a reminder that food is not just sustenance but a key player in the management of health conditions, a tool that, when used wisely, can support healing and well-being.

The Role of Protein: Quality Over Quantity

In the journey through Stage 5 Kidney Disease, the narrative around protein takes a pivotal turn. It's no longer a tale of simply piling on as much protein as possible but rather a thoughtful consideration of what kind of protein makes its way onto the plate. This shift from quantity to quality isn't just a minor plot twist in our dietary habits;

it's a fundamental change in how we view nutrition's role in managing a condition that profoundly affects every aspect of life.

Understanding Protein's Dual Role

Protein, the very foundation of our muscles and tissues, suddenly becomes a character with a complex backstory. Yes, it's essential, but in the context of advanced kidney disease, it's also a bit of a troublemaker. The body struggles to process the waste products from protein metabolism, turning what should be a straightforward nutritional requirement into a delicate balancing act.

Choosing Quality Over Quantity

The mantra 'more is better' fades away, replaced by the nuanced approach of 'better is more.' High-quality proteins, those rich in essential amino acids and easier for the body to use, take center stage. It's about finding those protein sources that give you the most bang for your buck, nutritionally speaking, without overburdening kidneys that are already working overtime.

Fish, chicken, eggs, and soy products become the heroes of this story, providing the body with the nutrients it needs without leaving behind a mess for the kidneys to clean up. It's a shift in perspective, seeing protein not just as a nutrient, but as a carefully chosen tool to support health.

The Rise of Plant-Based Proteins

And then there's the plot twist: plant-based proteins. Once relegated to the sidelines, they're now recognized for their starring role in a kidney-friendly diet. Beans, lentils, and nuts aren't just good for you; they're good for your kidneys, offering high-quality protein with a lower phosphorus footprint than their animal-based counterparts.

Embracing plant-based proteins isn't just about managing kidney disease; it's about opening up a whole new world of flavors and textures. It's a culinary adventure, one that invites creativity in the kitchen and brings a sense of joy and discovery to the dining table.

A Personal Journey

Determining the right amount and type of protein is deeply personal, a narrative that unfolds differently for everyone. It underscores the importance of a tailored approach, working hand in hand with healthcare professionals to craft a diet that supports not just kidney health but overall well-being.

This journey is about more than just following a set of dietary guidelines; it's about learning to listen to your body, understanding its needs, and responding with care and consideration. It's a process that fosters a deeper connection to food and a greater appreciation for its role in our health.

Reflecting on Protein's Role

As we reflect on the role of protein in managing Stage 5 Kidney Disease, it's clear that this is about more than just nutrition. It's about how we choose to nourish ourselves in the face of challenges, how we adapt and find resilience, and how we discover new ways to enjoy food and life despite the constraints we might face.

Reading Food Labels: What to Look For

Embarking on the journey of understanding food labels is akin to learning a new language. It's a skill that, once mastered, empowers us to make choices that can significantly impact our health and well-being, especially when navigating the complexities of Stage 5 Kidney Disease. This chapter isn't just about the mechanics of reading labels; it's an invitation to reflect on the profound relationship between the foods we consume and our health.

The Starting Point: Serving Sizes and Their Reality

The narrative of every food label begins with serving sizes and the number of servings per container. This information, often bypassed in our rush, is crucial. It grounds us in reality, reminding us that the portion we eat may not align with the 'serving size' defined by the manufacturer. Acknowledging this discrepancy is the first step towards mindful consumption, ensuring that what we eat supports our health goals and dietary needs.

The Critical Trio: Sodium, Potassium, and Phosphorus

For those of us managing Stage 5 Kidney Disease, three nutrients stand out on the label: sodium, potassium, and phosphorus. These elements, essential in moderation, become a focal point of our dietary management.

- **Sodium** lurks in many processed foods, and its presence on labels helps us steer toward choices that help maintain our blood pressure and fluid balance.

- **Potassium**, not always listed, is vital for heart and muscle function but must be consumed in careful amounts to avoid complications.

- **Phosphorus**, often hidden behind chemical names, requires a keen eye to identify and manage to protect our bones and hearts.

Understanding these nutrients' roles and managing their intake is not just about following dietary guidelines; it's about taking active steps to protect our kidney function and overall health.

Protein: More Than Just a Number

Protein content on labels is more than just a figure; it's a guide to selecting high-quality sources that meet our body's needs without overburdening our kidneys. This balance is not static but shifts based on individual health status and treatment plans, emphasizing the importance of personalized dietary advice.

Fats: Navigating the Landscape

Fats are not the enemy; rather, the type of fat matters. Food labels help us differentiate between the fats that support heart health and those we're better off minimizing. This distinction is particularly important for those of us with kidney disease, where cardiovascular health is a key concern.

Carbohydrates and Sugars: The Energy Providers

Carbohydrates are our body's primary energy source, but not all carbs are created equal. Food labels break down the total carbohydrates into dietary fiber and added sugars, offering insights into the food's nutritional value and its potential impact on our blood sugar levels. For those managing diabetes alongside kidney disease, this information is invaluable.

Ingredients: The Story Beyond the Numbers

The list of ingredients does more than detail what's in the food; it reveals the product's true nutritional story. This list, ordered by weight, helps us identify whole, nutritious foods versus those filled with additives and preservatives that might not serve our health.

Deciphering Claims: Seeing Through the Marketing

Claims like "low sodium" or "high fiber" are regulated, but they're also marketing tools. Understanding the standards behind these claims helps us make informed decisions, looking beyond the packaging to the true nutritional content of the food.

A Reflection on Empowerment

Learning to read food labels is a journey towards empowerment. It's about taking control of our dietary choices, making decisions that support our kidney health, and enhancing our overall well-being. It's a testament to the power of informed eating and a commitment to living well, even within the constraints of dietary restrictions.

CHAPTER 2

BREAKFAST RECIPES

Apple-Cinnamon Oatmeal

Prep Time: 5 mins

Total Time: 10 mins

Servings: 2

Ingredients

- 1 cup water
- ½ cup rolled oats
- 1 medium apple, peeled and diced
- ½ teaspoon cinnamon
- 1 tablespoon honey or maple syrup (optional)
- 2 tablespoons almond slices (optional)

Directions

1. Bring water to a boil in a small saucepan. Add oats and diced apple, reducing heat to a simmer.
2. Stir in cinnamon and honey or maple syrup if using. Cook until oats are soft and water is absorbed about 5 minutes.
3. Serve hot, garnished with almond slices for added texture and flavor.

Nutrition Facts (per serving)

- Calories: 150
- Fat: 2.5g

- Saturated Fat: 0.2g
- Cholesterol: 0mg
- Sodium: 10mg
- Carbohydrate: 29.5g
- Protein: 3g
- Phosphorus: 80mg
- Potassium: 115mg
- Fiber: 4g
- Calcium: 20mg

Low-Potassium Berry Smoothie

Prep Time: 5 mins
Total Time: 5 mins
Servings: 1
Ingredients
- 1 cup blueberries (fresh or frozen)
- ½ cup strawberries (fresh or frozen)
- 1 cup rice milk
- 1 tablespoon flaxseed meal

Directions
1. Combine blueberries, strawberries, rice milk, and flaxseed meal in a blender.
2. Blend on high until smooth, about 1 minute.
3. Serve immediately for a refreshing, low-potassium start to your day.

Nutrition Facts (per serving)
- Calories: 185
- Fat: 2.5g
- Saturated Fat: 0g
- Cholesterol: 0mg
- Sodium: 55mg
- Carbohydrate: 38g
- Protein: 3g
- Phosphorus: 65mg
- Potassium: 250mg
- Fiber: 7g
- Calcium: 30mg

Egg White Veggie Scramble

Prep Time: 5 mins
Total Time: 10 mins
Servings: 2
Ingredients
- 4 egg whites
- ½ cup diced bell peppers
- ¼ cup diced onions
- 1 cup spinach leaves
- 1 teaspoon olive oil
- Salt and pepper to taste

Directions
1. Heat olive oil in a non-stick skillet over medium heat. Sauté bell peppers and onions until soft, about 3 minutes.
2. Add spinach and cook until wilted about 2 minutes.
3. Pour egg whites over the vegetables, stirring gently. Cook until the egg whites are set, about 5 minutes. Season with salt and pepper.
4. Serve warm for a high-energy, low-protein breakfast.

Nutrition Facts (per serving)
- Calories: 90
- Fat: 2.5g
- Saturated Fat: 0.5g
- Cholesterol: 0mg
- Sodium: 170mg
- Carbohydrate: 5g
- Protein: 10g
- Phosphorus: 70mg
- Potassium: 220mg
- Fiber: 1g
- Calcium: 40mg

Avocado Toast with Radishes

Prep Time: 5 mins
Total Time: 5 mins
Servings: 2

Ingredients
- 2 slices whole grain bread, toasted
- 1 ripe avocado, mashed
- 4 radishes, thinly sliced
- Lemon juice, salt, and pepper to taste

Directions
1. Spread mashed avocado evenly on each slice of toasted bread.
2. Top with sliced radishes, then sprinkle with lemon juice, salt, and pepper to taste.
3. Serve immediately for a nutrient-rich, low-potassium breakfast option.

Nutrition Facts (per serving)
- Calories: 210
- Fat: 14g
- Saturated Fat: 2g
- Cholesterol: 0mg
- Sodium: 200mg
- Carbohydrate: 20g
- Protein: 5g
- Phosphorus: 100mg
- Potassium: 290mg
- Fiber: 7g
- Calcium: 20mg

Cottage Cheese with Pineapple

Prep Time: 2 mins

Total Time: 2 mins

Servings: 1

Ingredients

- ½ cup low-fat cottage cheese
- ½ cup pineapple chunks, in juice (drained)

Directions

1. Combine cottage cheese and pineapple chunks in a bowl.
2. Mix gently until the pineapple is evenly distributed through the cottage cheese.
3. Serve as a simple, nutritious starter or a light breakfast.

Nutrition Facts (per serving)

- Calories: 120
- Fat: 1g
- Saturated Fat: 0.5g
- Cholesterol: 5mg
- Sodium: 350mg
- Carbohydrate: 15g
- Protein: 12g
- Phosphorus: 150mg
- Potassium: 180mg
- Fiber: 1g
- Calcium: 100mg

Almond Butter Banana Smoothie

Prep Time: 5 mins
Total Time: 5 mins
Servings: 1

Ingredients
- 1 ripe banana
- 1 tablespoon almond butter
- 1 cup almond milk, unsweetened
- Ice cubes (optional)

Directions
1. Combine the banana, almond butter, almond milk, and ice cubes (if using) in a blender.
2. Blend until smooth and creamy.
3. Serve immediately for a refreshing and energizing breakfast.

Nutrition Facts (per serving)
- Calories: 210
- Fat: 10g
- Saturated Fat: 1g
- Cholesterol: 0mg
- Sodium: 180mg
- Carbohydrate: 27g
- Protein: 5g
- Phosphorus: 100mg
- Potassium: 422mg

- Fiber: 4g
- Calcium: 300mg

Chia Seed Pudding

Prep Time: 5 mins (plus overnight soaking)
Total Time: 8 hours 5 mins
Servings: 2
Ingredients
- ¼ cup chia seeds
- 1 cup coconut milk
- 1 tablespoon maple syrup
- ½ teaspoon vanilla extract
- Fresh berries for topping

Directions
1. In a bowl, mix chia seeds, coconut milk, maple syrup, and vanilla extract until well combined.
2. Cover and refrigerate overnight, or for at least 8 hours.
3. Stir the pudding, and add more coconut milk if it's too thick. Serve topped with fresh berries.

Nutrition Facts (per serving)
- Calories: 200
- Fat: 12g
- Saturated Fat: 5g
- Cholesterol: 0mg
- Sodium: 15mg
- Carbohydrate: 20g

- Protein: 4g
- Phosphorus: 150mg
- Potassium: 200mg
- Fiber: 8g
- Calcium: 250mg

Turkey and Spinach Omelet

Prep Time: 5 mins
Total Time: 10 mins
Servings: 1
Ingredients
- 2 egg whites
- ¼ cup cooked turkey breast, chopped
- ½ cup spinach, fresh
- 1 teaspoon olive oil
- Salt and pepper to taste

Directions
1. Heat olive oil in a skillet over medium heat. Sauté spinach until wilted, about 2 minutes.
2. In a bowl, whisk the egg whites with salt and pepper. Pour over the spinach into the skillet.
3. Add the chopped turkey breast. Cook until the eggs are set, fold the omelet in half, and serve.

Nutrition Facts (per serving)
- Calories: 150
- Fat: 5g

- Saturated Fat: 1g
- Cholesterol: 25mg
- Sodium: 200mg
- Carbohydrate: 2g
- Protein: 22g
- Phosphorus: 220mg
- Potassium: 300mg
- Fiber: 0.5g
- Calcium: 30mg

Quinoa Breakfast Bowl

Prep Time: 5 mins
Total Time: 20 mins
Servings: 2
Ingredients
- ½ cup quinoa, rinsed
- 1 cup water
- 1 apple, diced
- ½ teaspoon cinnamon
- 2 tablespoons walnuts, chopped
- Honey or maple syrup to taste

Directions
1. Combine quinoa and water in a saucepan. Bring to a boil, then cover and simmer for 15 minutes or until water is absorbed.

2. Stir in diced apple and cinnamon. Cook for another 2 minutes.
3. Serve in bowls, topped with chopped walnuts and a drizzle of honey or maple syrup.

Nutrition Facts (per serving)
- Calories: 235
- Fat: 8g
- Saturated Fat: 1g
- Cholesterol: 0mg
- Sodium: 10mg
- Carbohydrate: 36g
- Protein: 6g
- Phosphorus: 150mg
- Potassium: 320mg
- Fiber: 5g
- Calcium: 30mg

Ricotta and Honey Toast

Prep Time: 5 mins
Total Time: 5 mins
Servings: 2
Ingredients
- 2 slices whole grain bread, toasted
- ½ cup ricotta cheese
- 2 tablespoons honey
- A pinch of cinnamon (optional)

- Fresh figs or berries for topping (optional)

Directions
1. Spread ricotta cheese evenly over the toasted bread slices.
2. Drizzle honey over the ricotta and sprinkle with cinnamon if using.
3. Top with fresh figs or berries for added flavor and nutrition.

Nutrition Facts (per serving)
- Calories: 250
- Fat: 8g
- Saturated Fat: 5g
- Cholesterol: 30mg
- Sodium: 200mg
- Carbohydrate: 34g
- Protein: 12g
- Phosphorus: 180mg
- Potassium: 90mg
- Fiber: 2g
- Calcium: 200mg

CHAPTER 3

LUNCH RECIPES

Tuna Salad Stuffed Avocado

Prep Time: 10 mins
Total Time: 10 mins
Servings: 2

Ingredients

- 1 can (5 ounces) low-sodium tuna, drained
- 2 tablespoons mayonnaise
- 1 tablespoon lemon juice
- 1/4 cup diced celery
- 1/4 cup diced red bell pepper
- Salt and pepper to taste
- 2 avocados, halved and pitted
- Fresh parsley for garnish (optional)

Directions

1. In a bowl, mix the tuna, mayonnaise, lemon juice, celery, and red bell pepper. Season with salt and pepper to taste.
2. Spoon the tuna mixture into the avocado halves.
3. Garnish with fresh parsley if desired and serve immediately for a refreshing and satisfying lunch.

Nutrition Facts (per serving)

- Calories: 290
- Fat: 22g
- Saturated Fat: 3.5g
- Cholesterol: 30mg
- Sodium: 200mg
- Carbohydrate: 17g
- Protein: 12g
- Phosphorus: 150mg
- Potassium: 690mg
- Fiber: 7g
- Calcium: 30mg

Chickpea Greek Salad

Prep Time: 15 mins

Total Time: 15 mins

Servings: 4

Ingredients

- 2 cups canned chickpeas, rinsed and drained
- 1 cucumber, diced
- 1 cup cherry tomatoes, halved
- 1/2 cup diced red onion
- 1/4 cup chopped kalamata olives
- 1/4 cup crumbled feta cheese
- 2 tablespoons olive oil
- 1 tablespoon red wine vinegar

- 1 teaspoon dried oregano
- Salt and pepper to taste

Directions
1. In a large bowl, combine chickpeas, cucumber, cherry tomatoes, red onion, kalamata olives, and feta cheese.
2. In a small bowl, whisk together olive oil, red wine vinegar, oregano, salt, and pepper. Pour over the salad and toss to coat evenly.
3. Serve chilled or at room temperature for a refreshing and nutritious lunch.

Nutrition Facts (per serving)
- Calories: 250
- Fat: 12g
- Saturated Fat: 3g
- Cholesterol: 15mg
- Sodium: 300mg
- Carbohydrate: 27g
- Protein: 9g
- Phosphorus: 180mg
- Potassium: 360mg
- Fiber: 6g
- Calcium: 100mg

Vegetable Lentil Soup

Prep Time: 10 mins

Total Time: 40 mins

Servings: 4

Ingredients

- 1 tablespoon olive oil
- 1 onion, diced
- 2 carrots, diced
- 2 stalks celery, diced
- 2 cloves garlic, minced
- 1 cup dried lentils, rinsed
- 4 cups low-sodium vegetable broth
- 1 can (14.5 ounces) diced tomatoes, with juice
- 1 teaspoon dried thyme
- Salt and pepper to taste
- 2 cups baby spinach

Directions

1. Heat olive oil in a large pot over medium heat. Add onion, carrots, celery, and garlic; cook until softened, about 5 minutes.
2. Add lentils, vegetable broth, diced tomatoes with their juice, and thyme. Season with salt and pepper. Bring to a boil, then reduce heat and simmer, covered, until lentils are tender, about 30 minutes.

3. Stir in baby spinach and cook until wilted about 2 minutes. Serve hot for a warm, comforting meal.

Nutrition Facts (per serving)
- Calories: 240
- Fat: 4g
- Saturated Fat: 0.5g
- Cholesterol: 0mg
- Sodium: 300mg
- Carbohydrate: 38g
- Protein: 14g
- Phosphorus: 200mg
- Potassium: 710mg
- Fiber: 16g
- Calcium: 60mg

Quinoa Chicken Salad

Prep Time: 15 mins

Total Time: 15 mins (plus quinoa cooking time)

Servings: 4

Ingredients
- 2 cups cooked quinoa, cooled
- 1 cup cooked, shredded chicken breast
- 1 avocado, diced
- 1/2 cup cherry tomatoes, halved
- 1/4 cup diced cucumber
- 1/4 cup chopped cilantro

- 2 tablespoons lime juice
- 1 tablespoon olive oil
- Salt and pepper to taste

Directions
1. In a large bowl, combine quinoa, shredded chicken, avocado, cherry tomatoes, cucumber, and cilantro.
2. Drizzle with lime juice and olive oil, then season with salt and pepper. Toss to combine.
3. Serve chilled for a quick and easy lunch packed with protein and flavor.

Nutrition Facts (per serving)
- Calories: 290
- Fat: 13g
- Saturated Fat: 2g
- Cholesterol: 30mg
- Sodium: 70mg
- Carbohydrate: 27g
- Protein: 17g
- Phosphorus: 220mg
- Potassium: 520mg
- Fiber: 5g
- Calcium: 30mg

Turkey Wrap with Cranberry and Spinach

Prep Time: 5 mins
Total Time: 5 mins

Servings: 2

Ingredients
- 2 whole wheat tortillas
- 4 slices of low-sodium turkey breast
- 1/4 cup cranberry sauce
- 1 cup baby spinach leaves
- 1/4 cup shredded carrot

Directions
1. Lay out the tortillas and evenly spread cranberry sauce over each.
2. Layer turkey slices, spinach leaves, and shredded carrot on top of the cranberry sauce.
3. Roll up the tortillas tightly, cut them in half, and serve for a flavorful and nutritious lunch.

Nutrition Facts (per serving)
- Calories: 250
- Fat: 3g
- Saturated Fat: 0.5g
- Cholesterol: 25mg
- Sodium: 280mg
- Carbohydrate: 42g
- Protein: 15g
- Phosphorus: 100mg
- Potassium: 380mg
- Fiber: 5g
- Calcium: 40mg

Mediterranean Chickpea Salad

Prep Time: 15 mins

Total Time: 15 mins

Servings: 4

Ingredients
- 2 cups canned chickpeas, rinsed and drained
- 1 cup diced cucumbers
- 1 cup halved cherry tomatoes
- 1/2 cup diced red onion
- 1/4 cup chopped fresh parsley
- 1/4 cup crumbled feta cheese
- 2 tablespoons olive oil
- 1 tablespoon lemon juice
- Salt and pepper to taste

Directions
1. In a large bowl, combine chickpeas, cucumbers, cherry tomatoes, red onion, and parsley.
2. Add feta cheese, olive oil, and lemon juice. Season with salt and pepper to taste.
3. Toss everything together until well mixed. Serve chilled for a refreshing and nutritious Mediterranean-inspired lunch.

Nutrition Facts (per serving)
- Calories: 250
- Fat: 10g
- Saturated Fat: 3g

- Cholesterol: 15mg
- Sodium: 300mg
- Carbohydrate: 30g
- Protein: 10g
- Phosphorus: 180mg
- Potassium: 360mg
- Fiber: 8g
- Calcium: 120mg

Roasted Vegetable Quiche

Prep Time: 20 mins

Total Time: 1 hour

Servings: 6

Ingredients
- 1 pre-made pie crust
- 2 cups mixed vegetables (bell peppers, zucchini, and onions), roasted
- 4 eggs
- 1 cup low-fat milk
- 1/2 cup shredded low-fat cheese
- Salt and pepper to taste
- 1 teaspoon dried herbs (thyme or oregano)

Directions
1. Preheat oven to 375°F (190°C). Place the pie crust in a pie dish.
2. Spread the roasted vegetables evenly over the crust.

3. In a bowl, whisk together eggs, milk, cheese, salt, pepper, and dried herbs. Pour this mixture over the vegetables.
4. Bake for 40 minutes, or until the quiche is set and the crust is golden brown. Let cool for a few minutes before serving.

Nutrition Facts (per serving)
- Calories: 220
- Fat: 12g
- Saturated Fat: 4g
- Cholesterol: 140mg
- Sodium: 320mg
- Carbohydrate: 18g
- Protein: 10g
- Phosphorus: 190mg
- Potassium: 250mg
- Fiber: 2g
- Calcium: 150mg

Cold Pasta Salad with Tuna

Prep Time: 15 mins

Total Time: 15 mins (plus pasta cooking time)

Servings: 4

Ingredients
- 2 cups cooked whole wheat pasta, cooled
- 1 can (5 ounces) low-sodium tuna, drained and flaked
- 1 cup cherry tomatoes, halved
- 1/2 cup diced cucumber

- 1/4 cup sliced black olives
- 2 tablespoons chopped fresh basil
- 2 tablespoons olive oil
- 1 tablespoon red wine vinegar
- Salt and pepper to taste

Directions
1. In a large bowl, combine the cooked pasta, tuna, cherry tomatoes, cucumber, black olives, and fresh basil.
2. Drizzle with olive oil and red wine vinegar. Season with salt and pepper to taste.
3. Toss everything together until well combined. Chill in the refrigerator before serving for a cool and satisfying lunch.

Nutrition Facts (per serving)
- Calories: 280
- Fat: 10g
- Saturated Fat: 1.5g
- Cholesterol: 25mg
- Sodium: 200mg
- Carbohydrate: 32g
- Protein: 17g
- Phosphorus: 220mg
- Potassium: 300mg
- Fiber: 5g
- Calcium: 40mg

Chicken Avocado Wrap

Prep Time: 10 mins

Total Time: 10 mins

Servings: 2

Ingredients

- 2 whole wheat tortillas
- 1 cup cooked, shredded chicken breast
- 1 ripe avocado, mashed
- 1/2 cup shredded lettuce
- 1/4 cup diced tomatoes
- 2 tablespoons Greek yogurt
- Salt and pepper to taste

Directions

1. Spread the mashed avocado onto the center of each tortilla.
2. Top with shredded chicken, lettuce, and diced tomatoes.
3. Dollop Greek yogurt over the fillings, and season with salt and pepper.
4. Roll up the tortillas tightly, cut in half, and serve for a creamy and satisfying lunch.

Nutrition Facts (per serving)

- Calories: 350
- Fat: 15g
- Saturated Fat: 3g
- Cholesterol: 60mg
- Sodium: 320mg

- Carbohydrate: 32g
- Protein: 25g
- Phosphorus: 250mg
- Potassium: 500mg
- Fiber: 7g
- Calcium: 60mg

Beet and Goat Cheese Salad

Prep Time: 15 mins
Total Time: 15 mins
Servings: 4
Ingredients

- 4 cups mixed greens
- 1 cup cooked and sliced beets
- 1/2 cup crumbled goat cheese
- 1/4 cup walnuts, toasted
- 2 tablespoons balsamic vinegar
- 2 tablespoons olive oil
- Salt and pepper to taste

Directions

1. In a large bowl, combine mixed greens, sliced beets, goat cheese, and toasted walnuts.
2. In a small bowl, whisk together balsamic vinegar, olive oil, salt, and pepper.

3. Drizzle the dressing over the salad and toss gently to combine. Serve immediately for a vibrant and nutrient-rich lunch.

Nutrition Facts (per serving)
- Calories: 220
- Fat: 16g
- Saturated Fat: 4g
- Cholesterol: 13mg
- Sodium: 240mg
- Carbohydrate: 13g
- Protein: 7g
- Phosphorus: 120mg
- Potassium: 300mg
- Fiber: 3g
- Calcium: 60mg

CHAPTER 4

DINNER RECIPES

Baked Lemon Herb Chicken

Prep Time: 10 mins

Total Time: 40 mins

Servings: 4

Ingredients

- 4 boneless, skinless chicken breasts
- 2 tablespoons olive oil
- 1 lemon, juiced and zested
- 2 cloves garlic, minced
- 1 teaspoon dried thyme
- 1 teaspoon dried rosemary
- Salt and pepper to taste

Directions

1. Preheat oven to 375°F (190°C). In a small bowl, mix olive oil, lemon juice and zest, garlic, thyme, rosemary, salt, and pepper.
2. Place chicken breasts in a baking dish and pour the lemon herb mixture over them, ensuring each piece is well coated.
3. Bake in the preheated oven for 30 minutes, or until the chicken is cooked through and juices run clear.

4. Serve hot, garnished with lemon slices and additional fresh herbs if desired.

Nutrition Facts (per serving)
- Calories: 220
- Fat: 10g
- Saturated Fat: 1.5g
- Cholesterol: 65mg
- Sodium: 200mg
- Carbohydrate: 3g
- Protein: 29g
- Phosphorus: 250mg
- Potassium: 300mg
- Fiber: 0.5g
- Calcium: 20mg

One-Pot Vegetable Pasta

Prep Time: 10 mins
Total Time: 25 mins
Servings: 4
Ingredients
- 8 ounces whole wheat pasta
- 1 zucchini, sliced
- 1 bell pepper, diced
- 1 cup cherry tomatoes, halved
- 1 onion, diced
- 2 cloves garlic, minced

- 4 cups low-sodium vegetable broth
- 2 tablespoons olive oil
- Salt and pepper to taste
- Grated Parmesan cheese for serving (optional)

Directions

1. In a large pot, combine pasta, zucchini, bell pepper, cherry tomatoes, onion, garlic, vegetable broth, and olive oil. Season with salt and pepper.
2. Bring to a boil over high heat, then reduce to a simmer. Cook, stirring occasionally, until pasta is tender and most of the liquid has been absorbed, about 15 minutes.
3. Serve hot, garnished with grated Parmesan cheese if desired.

Nutrition Facts (per serving)

- Calories: 320
- Fat: 8g
- Saturated Fat: 1g
- Cholesterol: 0mg
- Sodium: 200mg
- Carbohydrate: 52g
- Protein: 10g
- Phosphorus: 150mg
- Potassium: 400mg
- Fiber: 8g
- Calcium: 30mg

Grilled Salmon with Dill Yogurt Sauce

Prep Time: 15 mins

Total Time: 25 mins

Servings: 4

Ingredients
- 4 salmon fillets (4 ounces each)
- 2 tablespoons olive oil
- Salt and pepper to taste
- 1 cup Greek yogurt
- 2 tablespoons fresh dill, chopped
- 1 tablespoon lemon juice
- 1 clove garlic, minced

Directions
1. Preheat the grill to medium-high heat. Brush salmon fillets with olive oil and season with salt and pepper.
2. Grill salmon for 5-6 minutes on each side, or until cooked through and easily flaked with a fork.
3. In a small bowl, mix Greek yogurt, dill, lemon juice, and garlic to make the sauce.
4. Serve grilled salmon with a dollop of dill yogurt sauce on top.

Nutrition Facts (per serving)
- Calories: 300
- Fat: 18g
- Saturated Fat: 3g

- Cholesterol: 60mg
- Sodium: 125mg
- Carbohydrate: 3g
- Protein: 29g
- Phosphorus: 350mg
- Potassium: 550mg
- Fiber: 0g
- Calcium: 80mg

Stuffed Bell Peppers

Prep Time: 20 mins

Total Time: 1 hr

Servings: 4

Ingredients

- 4 large bell peppers, tops removed and seeded
- 1 pound ground turkey
- 1 cup cooked quinoa
- 1 cup low-sodium tomato sauce
- 1 onion, diced
- 2 cloves garlic, minced
- 1 teaspoon dried oregano
- 1 teaspoon dried basil
- Salt and pepper to taste
- 1/2 cup shredded low-fat mozzarella cheese

Directions
1. Preheat oven to 350°F (175°C). In a skillet over medium heat, cook ground turkey, onion, and garlic until turkey is browned. Drain any excess fat.
2. Stir in cooked quinoa, tomato sauce, oregano, basil, salt, and pepper. Simmer for 5 minutes.
3. Stuff each bell pepper with the turkey and quinoa mixture. Place in a baking dish and cover with foil.
4. Bake for 45 minutes. Uncover, top each pepper with mozzarella cheese, and bake for an additional 15 minutes, or until the cheese is melted and bubbly.

Nutrition Facts (per serving)
- Calories: 350
- Fat: 12g
- Saturated Fat: 3g
- Cholesterol: 80mg
- Sodium: 300mg
- Carbohydrate: 32g
- Protein: 28g
- Phosphorus: 300mg
- Potassium: 700mg
- Fiber: 6g
- Calcium: 150mg

Roasted Chicken and Vegetables

Prep Time: 15 mins

Total Time: 1 hr 5 mins

Servings: 4

Ingredients

- 4 chicken thighs, bone-in and skin-on
- 2 carrots, sliced
- 2 parsnips, sliced
- 1 sweet potato, cubed
- 1 onion, quartered
- 2 tablespoons olive oil
- 1 teaspoon dried thyme
- Salt and pepper to taste

Directions

1. Preheat oven to 400°F (200°C). In a large roasting pan, toss carrots, parsnips, sweet potato, and onion with olive oil, thyme, salt, and pepper.
2. Place chicken thighs on top of the vegetables
3. . Season chicken with additional salt, pepper, and thyme.
4. Roast in the preheated oven for 50 minutes, or until chicken is golden and vegetables are tender.
5. Serve hot, ensuring a comforting and hearty meal that's both nutritious and satisfying.

Nutrition Facts (per serving)

- Calories: 410

- Fat: 22g
- Saturated Fat: 5g
- Cholesterol: 110mg
- Sodium: 220mg
- Carbohydrate: 33g
- Protein: 24g
- Phosphorus: 250mg
- Potassium: 800mg
- Fiber: 6g
- Calcium: 60mg

Herb-crusted cod with Asparagus

Prep Time: 10 mins
Total Time: 25 mins
Servings: 4
Ingredients

- 4 cod fillets (4 ounces each)
- 1 tablespoon olive oil
- 1 teaspoon lemon zest
- 2 tablespoons fresh parsley, finely chopped
- 1 tablespoon fresh dill, finely chopped
- Salt and pepper to taste
- 1 bunch asparagus, trimmed

Directions

1. Preheat oven to 400°F (200°C). Line a baking sheet with parchment paper.

2. Place cod fillets and asparagus on the baking sheet. Brush fillets with olive oil and season with lemon zest, parsley, dill, salt, and pepper.
3. Roast in the oven for 15 minutes, or until the cod is flaky and the asparagus is tender.
4. Serve immediately, offering a light yet flavorful dish perfect for any day of the week.

Nutrition Facts (per serving)
- Calories: 180
- Fat: 5g
- Saturated Fat: 1g
- Cholesterol: 60mg
- Sodium: 150mg
- Carbohydrate: 5g
- Protein: 28g
- Phosphorus: 250mg
- Potassium: 600mg
- Fiber: 2g
- Calcium: 50mg

Vegetarian Stuffed Zucchini Boats

Prep Time: 20 mins
Total Time: 40 mins
Servings: 4
Ingredients
- 4 medium zucchinis, halved lengthwise

- 1 cup cooked quinoa
- 1 can (15 ounces) low-sodium black beans, rinsed and drained
- 1 cup corn kernels, fresh or frozen
- 1/2 cup diced tomatoes
- 1 teaspoon cumin
- 1 teaspoon paprika
- Salt and pepper to taste
- 1/4 cup shredded low-fat cheese

Directions

1. Preheat oven to 375°F (190°C). Scoop out the center of each zucchini half to create a 'boat.'
2. In a bowl, mix quinoa, black beans, corn, diced tomatoes, cumin, paprika, salt, and pepper.
3. Fill each zucchini boat with the quinoa mixture. Top with shredded cheese.
4. Bake for 20 minutes, or until zucchini is tender and cheese is melted.
5. Serve warm, enjoying a hearty vegetarian option that doesn't skimp on flavor or nutrition.

Nutrition Facts (per serving)

- Calories: 220
- Fat: 4g
- Saturated Fat: 1g
- Cholesterol: 5mg
- Sodium: 200mg

- Carbohydrate: 36g
- Protein: 12g
- Phosphorus: 200mg
- Potassium: 700mg
- Fiber: 8g
- Calcium: 100mg

Lemon Garlic Shrimp with Broccoli

Prep Time: 10 mins
Total Time: 20 mins
Servings: 4
Ingredients

- 1 pound shrimp, peeled and deveined
- 2 tablespoons olive oil
- 3 cloves garlic, minced
- 1 lemon, juiced and zested
- 1 head broccoli, cut into florets
- Salt and pepper to taste

Directions

1. Heat olive oil in a large skillet over medium heat. Add garlic and cook until fragrant, about 1 minute.
2. Add shrimp, lemon juice, and zest to the skillet. Season with salt and pepper. Cook until shrimp are pink and opaque, about 5 minutes.
3. Steam broccoli until tender, about 5 minutes. Serve shrimp over steamed broccoli for a nutrient-rich, flavorful meal.

Nutrition Facts (per serving)

- Calories: 210
- Fat: 8g
- Saturated Fat: 1g
- Cholesterol: 180mg
- Sodium: 300mg
- Carbohydrate: 10g
- Protein: 25g
- Phosphorus: 250mg
- Potassium: 500mg
- Fiber: 4g
- Calcium: 100mg

Turkey and Sweet Potato Skillet

Prep Time: 10 mins

Total Time: 30 mins

Servings: 4

Ingredients

- 1 pound ground turkey
- 1 large sweet potato, cubed
- 1 onion, diced
- 2 cloves garlic, minced
- 1 teaspoon smoked paprika
- 1 teaspoon ground cumin
- Salt and pepper to taste
- 2 tablespoons olive oil

- 1/2 cup low-sodium chicken broth

Directions
1. Heat olive oil in a large skillet over medium heat. Add onion and garlic, cooking until softened.
2. Add ground turkey, breaking it apart with a spoon. Cook until browned.
3. Stir in sweet potato, smoked paprika, cumin, salt, and pepper. Add chicken broth and cover. Simmer until sweet potatoes are tender, about 15 minutes.
4. Serve hot, enjoying a comforting and nutritious one-pot meal that's easy to prepare.

Nutrition Facts (per serving)
- Calories: 320
- Fat: 12g
- Saturated Fat: 2g
- Cholesterol: 80mg
- Sodium: 200mg
- Carbohydrate: 24g
- Protein: 28g
- Phosphorus: 250mg
- Potassium: 650mg
- Fiber: 4g
- Calcium: 50mg

Grilled Vegetable Platter with Herb Drizzle

Prep Time: 15 mins

Total Time: 30 mins

Servings: 4

Ingredients

- 1 zucchini, sliced lengthwise
- 1 yellow squash, sliced lengthwise
- 1 red bell pepper, seeded and quartered
- 1 eggplant, sliced into rounds
- 2 tablespoons olive oil
- Salt and pepper to taste
- For the Herb Drizzle:
- 1/4 cup olive oil
- 2 tablespoons lemon juice
- 1 garlic clove, minced
- 2 tablespoons chopped fresh basil
- 1 tablespoon chopped fresh parsley
- Salt and pepper to taste

Directions

1. Preheat the grill to medium-high heat. Brush vegetables with olive oil and season with salt and pepper.
2. Grill vegetables, turning occasionally, until tender and charred, about 10-15 minutes.
3. For the herb drizzle, whisk together olive oil, lemon juice, garlic, basil, parsley, salt, and pepper in a small bowl.

4. Arrange grilled vegetables on a platter and drizzle with the herb mixture before serving. Enjoy a vibrant and nutritious dish perfect for any occasion.

Nutrition Facts (per serving)
- Calories: 210
- Fat: 14g
- Saturated Fat: 2g
- Cholesterol: 0mg
- Sodium: 75mg
- Carbohydrate: 20g
- Protein: 3g
- Phosphorus: 60mg
- Potassium: 450mg
- Fiber: 6g
- Calcium: 30mg

CHAPTER 5

SNACKS AND DESSERTS

Apple Cinnamon Chips

Prep Time: 10 mins

Total Time: 2 hrs 10 mins

Servings: 4

Ingredients

- 2 large apples, thinly sliced
- 1 teaspoon ground cinnamon

Directions

1. Preheat your oven to 200°F (93°C). Line a baking sheet with parchment paper.
2. Arrange apple slices in a single layer on the baking sheet. Sprinkle evenly with ground cinnamon.
3. Bake for 2 hours, flipping the slices halfway through until they are dry and crisp.
4. Let cool before serving as a crunchy, healthy snack.

Nutrition Facts (per serving)

- Calories: 65
- Fat: 0g
- Saturated Fat: 0g
- Cholesterol: 0mg
- Sodium: 2mg

- Carbohydrate: 17g
- Protein: 0.5g
- Phosphorus: 10mg
- Potassium: 134mg
- Fiber: 3g
- Calcium: 11mg

Rice Cake with Avocado and Tomato

Prep Time: 5 mins
Total Time: 5 mins
Servings: 1
Ingredients
- 1 plain rice cake
- 1/4 avocado, mashed
- 1/2 small tomato, sliced
- Salt and pepper to taste

Directions
1. Spread the mashed avocado onto the rice cake.
2. Top with sliced tomato and season with salt and pepper.
3. Serve immediately for a quick, nutritious snack that's both satisfying and kidney-friendly.

Nutrition Facts (per serving)
- Calories: 120
- Fat: 7g
- Saturated Fat: 1g
- Cholesterol: 0mg

- Sodium: 35mg
- Carbohydrate: 13g
- Protein: 2g
- Phosphorus: 52mg
- Potassium: 297mg
- Fiber: 4g
- Calcium: 12mg

Chilled Berry Soup

Prep Time: 10 mins

Total Time: 1 hr 10 mins (includes chilling)

Servings: 4

Ingredients

- 2 cups mixed berries (strawberries, blueberries, raspberries)
- 2 cups low-fat plain yogurt
- 2 tablespoons honey
- Mint leaves for garnish

Directions

1. In a blender, puree the mixed berries until smooth.
2. Strain the berry puree through a fine mesh sieve to remove seeds.
3. Whisk together the berry puree, yogurt, and honey until well combined.
4. Chill in the refrigerator for at least 1 hour.

5. Serve cold, garnished with mint leaves for a refreshing and guilt-free dessert.

Nutrition Facts (per serving)
- Calories: 150
- Fat: 2g
- Saturated Fat: 1g
- Cholesterol: 10mg
- Sodium: 70mg
- Carbohydrate: 28g
- Protein: 6g
- Phosphorus: 150mg
- Potassium: 250mg
- Fiber: 3g
- Calcium: 200mg

Peanut Butter Banana Bites

Prep Time: 15 mins

Total Time: 1 hr 15 mins (includes freezing)

Servings: 2

Ingredients
- 1 large banana
- 2 tablespoons natural peanut butter
- 1/4 cup dark chocolate chips, melted

Directions
1. Slice the banana into rounds.

2. Spread peanut butter on half of the slices and top with the remaining slices to make little banana sandwiches.
3. Dip each banana sandwich into melted dark chocolate, covering half of each bite.
4. Place on a baking sheet lined with parchment paper and freeze until the chocolate is set about 1 hour.
5. Enjoy a sweet treat without the guilt, perfect for a kidney-friendly diet.

Nutrition Facts (per serving)
- Calories: 200
- Fat: 11g
- Saturated Fat: 4g
- Cholesterol: 0mg
- Sodium: 75mg
- Carbohydrate: 24g
- Protein: 4g
- Phosphorus: 100mg
- Potassium: 322mg
- Fiber: 3g
- Calcium: 10mg

Vanilla Almond Mousse

Prep Time: 15 mins
Total Time: 1 hour 15 mins (includes chilling)
Servings: 4
Ingredients

- 1 cup low-fat cottage cheese
- 1/4 cup almond milk
- 2 tablespoons honey
- 1 teaspoon vanilla extract
- 1/4 cup sliced almonds, toasted

Directions

1. In a blender, combine cottage cheese, almond milk, honey, and vanilla extract until smooth.
2. Divide the mixture into serving dishes and chill in the refrigerator for at least 1 hour.
3. Before serving, sprinkle with toasted sliced almonds for added crunch and flavor.
4. Enjoy a creamy, low-sodium dessert that satisfies the sweet tooth in a kidney-friendly way.

Nutrition Facts (per serving)

- Calories: 120
- Fat: 4g
- Saturated Fat: 0.5g
- Cholesterol: 5mg
- Sodium: 200mg
- Carbohydrate: 13g
- Protein: 9g
- Phosphorus: 100mg
- Potassium: 150mg
- Fiber: 1g
- Calcium: 80mg

Cucumber Hummus Bites

Prep Time: 10 mins

Total Time: 10 mins

Servings: 4

Ingredients
- 2 large cucumbers, sliced into rounds
- 1 cup hummus
- Paprika for garnish
- Fresh parsley, chopped for garnish

Directions
1. Lay cucumber rounds on a serving platter.
2. Top each cucumber round with a spoonful of hummus.
3. Sprinkle with paprika and garnish with chopped parsley.
4. Serve immediately for a crisp, refreshing snack that's both nutritious and kidney-friendly.

Nutrition Facts (per serving)
- Calories: 150
- Fat: 9g
- Saturated Fat: 1.5g
- Cholesterol: 0mg
- Sodium: 200mg
- Carbohydrate: 13g
- Protein: 5g
- Phosphorus: 120mg
- Potassium: 310mg

- Fiber: 4g
- Calcium: 50mg

Carrot Cake Oatmeal Cookies

Prep Time: 15 mins
Total Time: 30 mins
Servings: 4
Ingredients

- 1 cup rolled oats
- 1/2 cup whole wheat flour
- 1/4 cup unsweetened applesauce
- 1/4 cup shredded carrots
- 2 tablespoons honey
- 1 teaspoon cinnamon
- 1/4 teaspoon nutmeg
- 1/4 cup raisins
- 1/4 cup chopped walnuts

Directions

1. Preheat oven to 350°F (175°C). Line a baking sheet with parchment paper.
2. In a large bowl, combine oats, flour, applesauce, shredded carrots, honey, cinnamon, and nutmeg. Mix until well combined.
3. Fold in raisins and walnuts.
4. Drop tablespoonfuls of the mixture onto the prepared baking sheet. Flatten slightly with the back of the spoon.

5. Bake for 15 minutes, or until edges are golden. Cool on a wire rack before serving.

Nutrition Facts (per serving)
- Calories: 220
- Fat: 8g
- Saturated Fat: 1g
- Cholesterol: 0mg
- Sodium: 25mg
- Carbohydrate: 34g
- Protein: 5g
- Phosphorus: 95mg
- Potassium: 270mg
- Fiber: 4g
- Calcium: 30mg

Frozen Yogurt Bark

Prep Time: 10 mins

Total Time: 2 hours 10 mins (includes freezing)

Servings: 4

Ingredients
- 2 cups low-fat Greek yogurt
- 2 tablespoons honey
- 1/2 cup mixed berries (strawberries, blueberries)
- 1/4 cup sliced almonds

Directions

1. Mix Greek yogurt with honey in a bowl. Spread the mixture evenly onto a baking sheet lined with parchment paper.
2. Sprinkle mixed berries and sliced almonds over the yogurt.
3. Freeze for at least 2 hours until firm. Break into pieces and serve as a frozen treat.

Nutrition Facts (per serving)

- Calories: 180
- Fat: 5g
- Saturated Fat: 0.5g
- Cholesterol: 10mg
- Sodium: 50mg
- Carbohydrate: 20g
- Protein: 15g
- Phosphorus: 150mg
- Potassium: 240mg
- Fiber: 2g
- Calcium: 150mg

Zucchini Bread Muffins

Prep Time: 15 mins

Total Time: 35 mins

Servings: 6

Ingredients

- 1 cup whole wheat flour

- 1/2 cup almond flour
- 1/4 cup honey
- 1 teaspoon baking powder
- 1/2 teaspoon cinnamon
- 1/4 teaspoon nutmeg
- 2 eggs, beaten
- 1 cup grated zucchini
- 1/4 cup unsweetened applesauce
- 1 teaspoon vanilla extract

Directions

1. Preheat oven to 350°F (175°C). Line a muffin tin with paper liners.
2. In a large bowl, mix whole wheat flour, almond flour, honey, baking powder, cinnamon, and nutmeg.
3. Stir in eggs, grated zucchini, applesauce, and vanilla extract until well combined.
4. Divide the batter evenly among the muffin cups.
5. Bake for 20 minutes, or until a toothpick inserted into the center comes out clean.
6. Cool on a wire rack before serving. Enjoy a moist, flavorful muffin that's perfect for a guilt-free snack or dessert.

Nutrition Facts (per serving)

- Calories: 180
- Fat: 6g
- Saturated Fat: 1g
- Cholesterol: 62mg

- Sodium: 80mg
- Carbohydrate: 27g
- Protein: 7g
- Phosphorus: 120mg
- Potassium: 200mg
- Fiber: 3g
- Calcium: 60mg

Peach Sorbet

Prep Time: 10 mins

Total Time: 2 hours 10 mins (includes freezing)

Servings: 4

Ingredients

- 4 cups frozen peaches
- 1/4 cup honey
- 1/2 cup water
- 1 tablespoon lemon juice

Directions

1. In a blender, combine frozen peaches, honey, water, and lemon juice. Blend until smooth.
2. Pour the mixture into a freezer-safe container and freeze until solid, about 2 hours.
3. Before serving, let the sorbet sit at room temperature for a few minutes to soften slightly.
4. Serve as a refreshing, low-potassium dessert that's both sweet and satisfying.

Nutrition Facts (per serving)
- Calories: 160
- Fat: 0g
- Saturated Fat: 0g
- Cholesterol: 0mg
- Sodium: 5mg
- Carbohydrate: 40g
- Protein: 2g
- Phosphorus: 30mg
- Potassium: 330mg
- Fiber: 3g
- Calcium: 10mg

CHAPTER 6

BEVERAGES AND SMOOTHIES

Cucumber Mint Water

Prep Time: 5 mins

Total Time: 1 hour 5 mins (includes chilling)

Servings: 4

Ingredients

- 1 large cucumber, thinly sliced
- 10 mint leaves, roughly torn
- 4 cups water

Directions

1. In a large pitcher, combine cucumber slices, mint leaves, and water.
2. Stir gently to mix. Refrigerate for at least 1 hour to allow flavors to infuse.
3. Serve chilled for a refreshing and hydrating beverage that's perfect for kidney health.

Nutrition Facts (per serving)

- Calories: 0
- Fat: 0g
- Saturated Fat: 0g
- Cholesterol: 0mg
- Sodium: 0mg

- Carbohydrate: 0g
- Protein: 0g
- Phosphorus: 0mg
- Potassium: 76mg (varies based on cucumber content)
- Fiber: 0g
- Calcium: 0mg

Berry Blast Kidney-Friendly Smoothie

Prep Time: 5 mins
Total Time: 5 mins
Servings: 2

Ingredients
- 1 cup fresh strawberries, hulled
- 1/2 cup blueberries
- 1 banana, sliced
- 1 cup almond milk, unsweetened
- Ice cubes (optional)

Directions
1. In a blender, combine strawberries, blueberries, banana, and almond milk. Add ice cubes if a colder smoothie is desired.
2. Blend on high until smooth and creamy.
3. Serve immediately for a nutrient-rich smoothie that's low in potassium and phosphorus, making it a great choice for those with kidney concerns.

Nutrition Facts (per serving)
- Calories: 120

- Fat: 1.5g
- Saturated Fat: 0g
- Cholesterol: 0mg
- Sodium: 80mg
- Carbohydrate: 26g
- Protein: 2g
- Phosphorus: 50mg
- Potassium: 322mg
- Fiber: 4g
- Calcium: 150mg

Chamomile Lavender Tea

Prep Time: 5 mins
Total Time: 10 mins
Servings: 2
Ingredients
- 2 chamomile tea bags
- 1 teaspoon dried lavender flowers
- 2 cups boiling water

Directions
1. Place chamomile tea bags and dried lavender flowers in a teapot.
2. Pour boiling water over the tea bags and lavender. Cover and steep for 5 minutes.

3. Strain into cups and serve hot. Enjoy a calming beverage that's beneficial for relaxation and hydration, suitable for those managing kidney disease.

Nutrition Facts (per serving)
- Calories: 0
- Fat: 0g
- Saturated Fat: 0g
- Cholesterol: 0mg
- Sodium: 0mg
- Carbohydrate: 0g
- Protein: 0g
- Phosphorus: 0mg
- Potassium: 0mg
- Fiber: 0g
- Calcium: 0mg

Green Detox Smoothie

Prep Time: 5 mins
Total Time: 5 mins
Servings: 2
Ingredients
- 1 cup fresh spinach leaves
- 1/2 cucumber, sliced
- 1 green apple, cored and sliced
- 1 tablespoon lemon juice
- 1 cup coconut water

Directions

1. In a blender, combine spinach, cucumber, green apple, lemon juice, and coconut water.
2. Blend on high until smooth. Add water to adjust consistency if necessary.
3. Serve immediately for a detoxifying smoothie that supports kidney health with its low potassium and phosphorus content.

Nutrition Facts (per serving)

- Calories: 60
- Fat: 0.5g
- Saturated Fat: 0g
- Cholesterol: 0mg
- Sodium: 25mg
- Carbohydrate: 14g
- Protein: 1g
- Phosphorus: 20mg
- Potassium: 200mg
- Fiber: 2g
- Calcium: 30mg

Ginger Pear Infusion

Prep Time: 5 mins

Total Time: 1 hour 5 mins (includes infusing)

Servings: 4

Ingredients

- 1 pear, thinly sliced
- 1-inch piece of ginger, thinly sliced
- 4 cups water

Directions

1. In a large pitcher, combine pear slices, ginger slices, and water.
2. Refrigerate for at least 1 hour to allow the flavors to infuse into the water.
3. Serve chilled for a subtly sweet and refreshing drink that's both hydrating and kidney-friendly.

Nutrition Facts (per serving)

- Calories: 0 (minimal from pear)
- Fat: 0g
- Saturated Fat: 0g
- Cholesterol: 0mg
- Sodium: 0mg
- Carbohydrate: 0g (minimal from pear)
- Protein: 0g
- Phosphorus: 0mg
- Potassium: 0mg (varies based on pear content)
- Fiber: 0g
- Calcium: 0mg

Watermelon Cucumber Slush

Prep Time: 10 mins
Total Time: 10 mins

Servings: 2

Ingredients
- 2 cups cubed seedless watermelon, frozen
- 1 small cucumber, peeled and sliced
- Juice of 1 lime
- 1 tablespoon honey (optional)
- Mint leaves for garnish

Directions
1. In a blender, combine frozen watermelon cubes, cucumber slices, lime juice, and honey if desired. Blend until smooth and slushy.
2. Pour into glasses and garnish with mint leaves. Serve immediately for a refreshing and hydrating drink that's perfect for warm days.

Nutrition Facts (per serving)
- Calories: 80
- Fat: 0g
- Saturated Fat: 0g
- Cholesterol: 0mg
- Sodium: 2mg
- Carbohydrate: 20g
- Protein: 1g
- Phosphorus: 15mg
- Potassium: 270mg
- Fiber: 1g
- Calcium: 20mg

Almond Milk Matcha Latte

Prep Time: 5 mins

Total Time: 5 mins

Servings: 1

Ingredients
- 1 teaspoon matcha green tea powder
- 1 tablespoon hot water
- 1 cup unsweetened almond milk, warmed
- Honey or sweetener of choice, to taste

Directions
1. In a cup, whisk together matcha powder and hot water until smooth.
2. Warm the almond milk in a saucepan or microwave, then pour it into the cup with the matcha mixture.
3. Sweeten with honey or your preferred sweetener to taste. Stir well and serve warm for a cozy, antioxidant-rich beverage.

Nutrition Facts (per serving)
- Calories: 40
- Fat: 3g
- Saturated Fat: 0g
- Cholesterol: 0mg
- Sodium: 180mg
- Carbohydrate: 2g
- Protein: 1g

- Phosphorus: 20mg
- Potassium: 50mg
- Fiber: 1g
- Calcium: 300mg

Pineapple Coconut Water Smoothie

Prep Time: 5 mins
Total Time: 5 mins
Servings: 2

Ingredients
- 1 cup pineapple chunks, fresh or frozen
- 1 cup coconut water
- 1/2 banana, sliced
- Ice cubes (optional)

Directions
1. In a blender, combine pineapple chunks, coconut water, banana, and ice cubes if desired.
2. Blend until smooth and creamy.
3. Serve immediately for a tropical, hydrating smoothie that's low in potassium and gentle on the kidneys.

Nutrition Facts (per serving)
- Calories: 70
- Fat: 0g
- Saturated Fat: 0g
- Cholesterol: 0mg
- Sodium: 42mg

- Carbohydrate: 18g
- Protein: 1g
- Phosphorus: 10mg
- Potassium: 200mg
- Fiber: 2g
- Calcium: 30mg

Herbal Berry Iced Tea

Prep Time: 5 mins

Total Time: 1 hour 5 mins (includes cooling)

Servings: 4

Ingredients

- 4 cups water
- 2 herbal berry tea bags
- 1/4 cup fresh berries (strawberries, blueberries)
- Honey or sweetener of choice, to taste
- Ice cubes

Directions

1. Boil water and steep the herbal berry tea bags for 5 minutes. Remove the tea bags and let the tea cool.
2. Once cooled, sweeten the tea with honey or your preferred sweetener to taste.
3. Add fresh berries to a pitcher, pour the cooled tea over them, and add ice cubes.
4. Chill in the refrigerator or serve immediately for a refreshing and kidney-friendly beverage.

Nutrition Facts (per serving)

- Calories: 10
- Fat: 0g
- Saturated Fat: 0g
- Cholesterol: 0mg
- Sodium: 0mg
- Carbohydrate: 3g
- Protein: 0g
- Phosphorus: 0mg
- Potassium: 15mg
- Fiber: 1g
- Calcium: 0mg

Golden Milk Turmeric Tea

Prep Time: 5 mins
Total Time: 10 mins
Servings: 1
Ingredients

- 1 cup almond milk
- 1 teaspoon turmeric powder
- 1/2 teaspoon cinnamon
- 1/4 teaspoon ginger powder
- Honey or sweetener of choice, to taste

Directions

1. In a small saucepan, heat the almond milk over medium heat.

2. Whisk in turmeric, cinnamon, and ginger powder until well combined.
3. Heat the mixture until warm but not boiling. Sweeten with honey or your preferred sweetener to taste.
4. Serve warm for a comforting beverage full of anti-inflammatory benefits, perfect for a relaxing evening.

Nutrition Facts (per serving)
- Calories: 60
- Fat: 2.5g
- Saturated Fat: 0g
- Cholesterol: 0mg
- Sodium: 180mg
- Carbohydrate: 8g
- Protein: 1g
- Phosphorus: 0mg
- Potassium: 50mg
- Fiber: 1g
- Calcium: 300mg

CHAPTER 7

MEAL PLAN

Day 1
- **Breakfast:** Apple-Cinnamon Oatmeal
- **Lunch:** Tuna Salad Stuffed Avocado
- **Dinner:** Baked Lemon Herb Chicken with Asparagus
- **Snacks/Beverages:** Cucumber Mint Water, Apple Cinnamon Chips

Day 2
- **Breakfast:** Low-Potassium Berry Smoothie
- **Lunch:** Chickpea Greek Salad
- **Dinner:** One-Pot Vegetable Pasta
- **Snacks/Beverages:** Rice Cake with Avocado and Tomato, Chamomile Lavender Tea

Day 3
- **Breakfast:** Egg White Veggie Scramble
- **Lunch:** Vegetable Lentil Soup
- **Dinner:** Grilled Salmon with Dill Yogurt Sauce
- **Snacks/Beverages:** Herbal Berry Iced Tea, Peanut Butter Banana Bites

Day 4

- **Breakfast:** Avocado Toast with Radishes
- **Lunch:** Quinoa Chicken Salad
- **Dinner:** Stuffed Bell Peppers
- **Snacks/Beverages:** Green Detox Smoothie, Frozen Yogurt Bark

Day 5

- **Breakfast:** Cottage Cheese with Pineapple
- **Lunch:** Turkey Wrap with Cranberry and Spinach
- **Dinner:** Roasted Chicken and Vegetables
- **Snacks/Beverages:** Watermelon Cucumber Slush, Zucchini Bread Muffins

Day 6

- **Breakfast:** Berry Blast Kidney-Friendly Smoothie
- **Lunch:** Mediterranean Chickpea Salad
- **Dinner:** Herb-Crusted Cod with Asparagus
- **Snacks/Beverages:** Almond Milk Matcha Latte, Carrot Cake Oatmeal Cookies

Day 7

- **Breakfast:** Chia Seed Pudding
- **Lunch:** Roasted Vegetable Quiche
- **Dinner:** Lemon Garlic Shrimp with Broccoli
- **Snacks/Beverages:** Pineapple Coconut Water Smoothie, Cucumber Hummus Bites

Day 8
- **Breakfast:** Quinoa Breakfast Bowl
- **Lunch:** Cold Pasta Salad with Tuna
- **Dinner:** Turkey and Sweet Potato Skillet
- **Snacks/Beverages:** Ginger Pear Infusion, Vanilla Almond Mousse

Day 9
- **Breakfast:** Ricotta and Honey Toast
- **Lunch:** Chicken Avocado Wrap
- **Dinner:** Balsamic Glazed Salmon
- **Snacks/Beverages:** Peach Sorbet, Chamomile Lavender Tea

Day 10
- **Breakfast:** Almond Butter Banana Smoothie
- **Lunch:** Beet and Goat Cheese Salad
- **Dinner:** Grilled Vegetable Platter with Herb Drizzle
- **Snacks/Beverages:** Golden Milk Turmeric Tea, Apple Cinnamon Chips

Day 11
- **Breakfast:** Berry Blast Kidney-Friendly Smoothie
- **Lunch:** Turkey and Sweet Potato Skillet
- **Dinner:** Grilled Vegetable Platter with Herb Drizzle
- **Snack:** Cucumber Hummus Bites

Day 12

- **Breakfast:** Chia Seed Pudding
- **Lunch:** Quinoa Chicken Salad
- **Dinner:** Lemon Garlic Shrimp with Broccoli
- **Snack:** Apple Cinnamon Chips

Day 13

- **Breakfast:** Rice Cake with Avocado and Tomato
- **Lunch:** Mediterranean Chickpea Salad
- **Dinner:** Balsamic Glazed Salmon
- **Snack:** Carrot Cake Oatmeal Cookies

Day 14

- **Breakfast:** Quinoa Breakfast Bowl
- **Lunch:** Cold Pasta Salad with Tuna
- **Dinner:** Mushroom and Barley Soup
- **Snack:** Frozen Yogurt Bark

Day 15

- **Breakfast:** Almond Butter Banana Smoothie
- **Lunch:** Vegetarian Stuffed Zucchini Boats
- **Dinner:** Soy-glazed chicken with Steamed Greens
- **Snack:** Peach Sorbet

Day 16

- **Breakfast:** Vanilla Almond Mousse
- **Lunch:** Chicken Avocado Wrap

- **Dinner:** Grilled Salmon with Dill Yogurt Sauce
- **Snack:** Watermelon Cucumber Slush

Day 17

- **Breakfast:** Cucumber Mint Water
- **Lunch:** Beet and Goat Cheese Salad
- **Dinner:** Stuffed Bell Peppers
- **Snack:** Pineapple Coconut Water Smoothie

Day 18

- **Breakfast:** Herbal Berry Iced Tea
- **Lunch:** Turkey Wrap with Cranberry and Spinach
- **Dinner:** Roasted Chicken and Vegetables
- **Snack:** Zucchini Bread Muffins

Day 19

- **Breakfast:** Golden Milk Turmeric Tea
- **Lunch:** Chickpea Greek Salad
- **Dinner:** Herb-Crusted Cod with Asparagus
- **Snack:** Ginger Pear Infusion

Day 20

- **Breakfast:** Apple-Cinnamon Oatmeal
- **Lunch:** One-Pot Vegetable Pasta
- **Dinner:** Chamomile Lavender Tea
- **Snack:** Peanut Butter Banana Bites

Day 21
- **Breakfast:** Low-Potassium Berry Smoothie
- **Lunch:** Roasted Vegetable Quiche
- **Dinner:** Almond Milk Matcha Latte
- **Snack:** Green Detox Smoothie

Day 22
- **Breakfast:** Egg White Veggie Scramble
- **Lunch:** Lentil and Spinach Curry
- **Dinner:** Quinoa Stuffed Bell Peppers
- **Snack:** Rice Cake with Avocado and Tomato

Day 23
- **Breakfast:** Avocado Toast with Radishes
- **Lunch:** Cold Pasta Salad with Tuna
- **Dinner:** Baked Lemon Herb Chicken
- **Snack:** Apple Cinnamon Chips

Day 24
- **Breakfast:** Cottage Cheese with Pineapple
- **Lunch:** Mediterranean Chickpea Salad
- **Dinner:** Lemon Garlic Shrimp with Broccoli
- **Snack:** Carrot Cake Oatmeal Cookies

Day 25
- **Breakfast:** Berry Blast Kidney-Friendly Smoothie
- **Lunch:** Turkey and Sweet Potato Skillet

- **Dinner:** Grilled Vegetable Platter with Herb Drizzle
- **Snack:** Cucumber Hummus Bites

Day 26

- **Breakfast:** Chia Seed Pudding
- **Lunch:** Quinoa Chicken Salad
- **Dinner:** Balsamic Glazed Salmon
- **Snack:** Frozen Yogurt Bark

Day 27

- **Breakfast:** Rice Cake with Avocado and Tomato
- **Lunch:** Vegetarian Stuffed Zucchini Boats
- **Dinner:** Soy-glazed chicken with Steamed Greens
- **Snack:** Peach Sorbet

Day 28

- **Breakfast:** Quinoa Breakfast Bowl
- **Lunch:** Cold Pasta Salad with Tuna
- **Dinner:** Mushroom and Barley Soup
- **Snack:** Zucchini Bread Muffins

Day 29

- **Breakfast:** Almond Butter Banana Smoothie
- **Lunch:** Chicken Avocado Wrap
- **Dinner:** Grilled Salmon with Dill Yogurt Sauce
- **Snack:** Watermelon Cucumber Slush

Day 30
- **Breakfast:** Vanilla Almond Mousse
- **Lunch:** Beet and Goat Cheese Salad
- **Dinner:** Stuffed Bell Peppers
- **Snack:** Pineapple Coconut Water Smoothie

Frequently asked questions

Stage 5 Kidney Disease, also known as End-Stage Renal Disease (ESRD), raises numerous questions for patients and their families. Here are some frequently asked questions about this condition:

1. What is Stage 5 Kidney Disease?

Stage 5 Kidney Disease is the final stage of chronic kidney disease (CKD), characterized by severe loss of kidney function. At this stage, the kidneys are unable to perform their essential functions effectively, such as filtering waste and excess fluids from the blood.

2. What causes Stage 5 Kidney Disease?

The leading causes of Stage 5 Kidney Disease include diabetes and high blood pressure, which can damage the kidneys over time. Other causes may include chronic glomerulonephritis, polycystic kidney disease, prolonged obstruction of the urinary tract, and certain autoimmune diseases.

3. What are the symptoms of Stage 5 Kidney Disease?

Symptoms may include nausea, vomiting, fatigue, weakness, sleep problems, changes in urine output, decreased mental sharpness, muscle cramps, swelling of feet and ankles, persistent itching, and chest pain.

4. How is Stage 5 Kidney Disease diagnosed?

Diagnosis typically involves blood tests to measure creatinine levels and calculate glomerular filtration rate (GFR), urine tests to check for protein or blood, imaging tests to assess kidney structure, and sometimes a kidney biopsy to determine the specific type of kidney damage.

5. What treatment options are available for Stage 5 Kidney Disease?

Treatment options include dialysis (hemodialysis or peritoneal dialysis) to remove waste products and excess fluid from the blood, and kidney transplantation, which involves replacing the diseased kidneys with a healthy kidney from a donor.

6. Can diet and lifestyle changes help manage Stage 5 Kidney Disease?

Yes, diet and lifestyle changes are crucial in managing Stage 5 Kidney Disease. These may include a low-protein, low-salt, and low-potassium diet, fluid restrictions, and avoiding substances that can further damage the kidneys. Consulting with a renal dietitian is essential for personalized dietary guidance.

7. How does Stage 5 Kidney Disease affect daily life?

The impact on daily life can be significant, with changes in diet, the need for regular dialysis treatments, and managing symptoms. It can also affect emotional well-being, requiring support from healthcare providers, family, and support groups.

8. Is kidney transplantation a cure for Stage 5 Kidney Disease?

While a successful kidney transplant can restore normal kidney function, it is not considered a cure. Recipients need to take immunosuppressive medications for the rest of their lives to prevent organ rejection, and there's always a risk of complications.

9. How can I support a loved one with Stage 5 Kidney Disease?

Support can include helping with treatment management, attending medical appointments, making dietary adjustments, offering emotional support, and encouraging participation in support groups for both patients and caregivers.

10. What is the prognosis for someone with Stage 5 Kidney Disease?

The prognosis varies widely depending on factors like the underlying cause, overall health, age, and how well the patient responds to treatment. Dialysis and kidney transplantation can significantly improve quality of life and life expectancy.

CHAPTER 8

CONCLUSION

As we conclude our journey through the "Stage 5 Kidney Disease Diet Cookbook for Seniors," it's important to reflect on the path we've traversed together. Journeying the complexities of kidney disease, especially at Stage 5, is no small feat. It requires courage, resilience, and an unwavering commitment to your health and well-being. This cookbook has been more than just a collection of recipes; it's been a guide, a companion, and a source of hope in managing a condition that affects every aspect of life.

Understanding and managing Stage 5 Kidney Disease is a profound challenge, one that you face daily with strength and grace. Dietary adjustments and lifestyle changes are significant, but they are also powerful tools for maintaining your quality of life and health. Each recipe in this cookbook has been crafted with your needs in mind, focusing on kidney-friendly ingredients while never compromising on flavor or the joy of eating.

It's natural to feel overwhelmed at times, given the restrictions and the need for careful management of your diet. However, remember that each step you take, no matter how small, is a victory. Every mindful choice you make about what to eat, every time you choose a kidney-friendly meal over an easier, less healthy option, you are taking control of your health and your life. These decisions are acts of self-care and self-respect.

The journey with Stage 5 Kidney Disease is undoubtedly challenging, but it's also filled with opportunities for growth, learning, and deepening connections with those who support you. Embracing a diet that supports your kidney health can open new doors to understanding nutrition, exploring new flavors, and enjoying meals that nourish both your body and soul. This cookbook aims to be a beacon of light, guiding you toward choices that enhance your well-being.

To the caregivers, family members, and friends who stand by those managing kidney disease, your role is invaluable. Your support, understanding, and willingness to adapt alongside your loved ones make a world of difference. Together, you can navigate the challenges, celebrate the successes, and enjoy the journey of discovery that comes with adapting to a kidney-friendly diet.

As you continue on this path, remember that you are not alone. A community of individuals and families are on similar journeys, facing the same challenges and celebrating similar victories. Lean on these connections, share your experiences, and draw strength from the knowledge that your journey contributes to a collective understanding and management of kidney disease.

In moments of doubt or difficulty, remind yourself of the strength that has carried you this far. The resilience you've shown in the face of adversity is a testament to your spirit and determination. Let this cookbook serve not just as a guide to kidney-friendly cooking but as a reminder of your capability to adapt and thrive, even in the face of challenges.

As you move forward, let the lessons learned and the joy found in each recipe inspire you to continue making choices that support your health and happiness. Your journey is unique, and your strength is immense. With each day, with every meal, you are taking steps towards a healthier, more vibrant life.

In closing, I leave you with a motivational quote that encapsulates the spirit of resilience and hope: "*The human spirit is stronger than anything that can happen to it.*" – C.C. Scott. This quote reminds us that despite the challenges of Stage 5 Kidney Disease, your spirit, your will to persevere, and your capacity for joy are indomitable. May you carry this strength with you, in every choice you make, in every meal you prepare, and in every moment you cherish.

www.ingramcontent.com/pod-product-compliance
Lightning Source LLC
Chambersburg PA
CBHW050322230526
45471CB00005B/2313